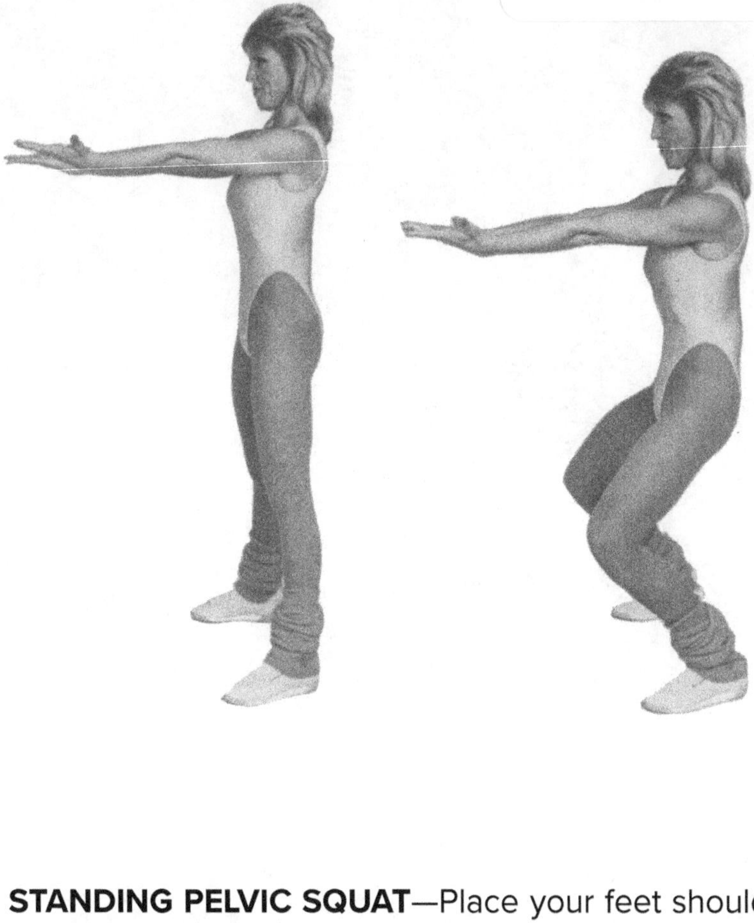

2. STANDING PELVIC SQUAT—Place your feet shoulder width apart, and bend your knees. Pulse up and down only¼ of the way. Have your arms out straight with the palms facing upward. Move up and down for approximately 1 minute.

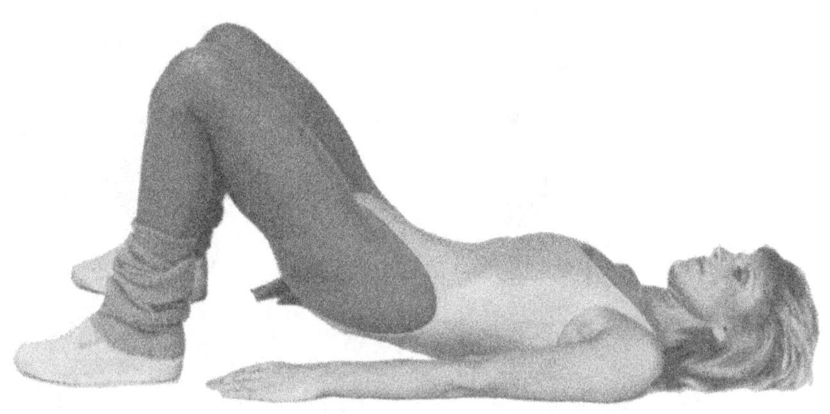

12 MINUTES TO: FIRM FANNIES

by JOANIE GREGGAINS

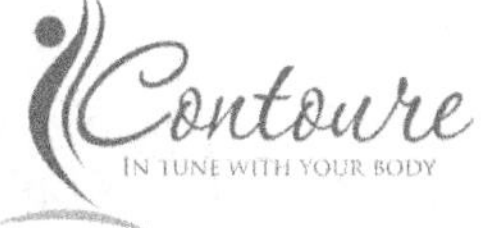

Use your phone or tablet to scan the QR code and click on the URL to listen to the Word-for-Word Audio Read-Along.

Congratulations FITNESS FANS

You are only 12 MINUTES away from having

FIRMER FANNYS

We all know that the gluteal muscles are one of the largest muscle groups in the body. Of all the muscle groups gravity seems to affect the gluteals the most. That's right, we've all noticed that downward slide. Well don't despair, because this work out is going to Strengthen, Firm, Lift, and Reduce those muscles. You're going to look great in those jeans. You'll never worry about turning your back on any one again. Good bye double bubble.

But, the benefits of this work out go beyond having Firmer Fannys. You will improve your circulation, increase your vitality, and replace fat with muscle.

So put on this recording and let's get started.

Remember, do what you can. Don't worry , if you can't do all of the repetitions. One way that you'll realize the results of this program, is that in a few weeks you'll be able to do more repetitions. This is one of the ways that you'll be able to see your improvement.

So, let's get started!

Make sure that you have enough room for your lifts. Also, wear loose clothing, and exercise on a mat or a soft carpet.

Before you begin any exercise program you should consult your physician.

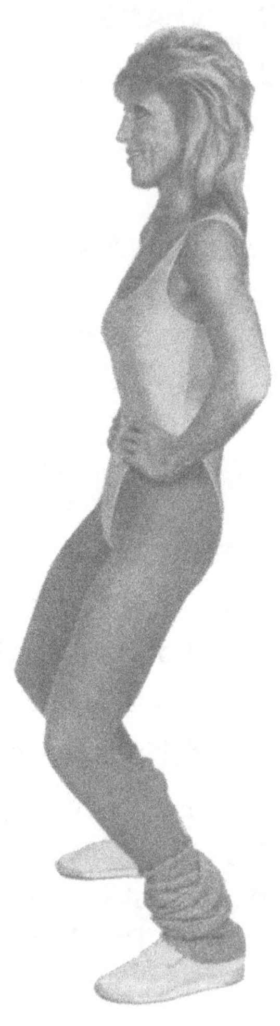

1. STANDING PELVIC ROLL—Stand with the feet apart and your toes forward. Keep the knees bent and bring the hips forward and then upward. Hold the stomach in and press with the gluteals. Do this with a rocking motion for approximately 1 minute.

3. (Now go down to the floor, and press your back flat against the floor.)

4. BASIC PELVIC TILT—Keep your back flat on the floor, and bend your knees while keeping your feet flat on the floor. Lift the gluteals. Press off the heels and lift your pelvic area towards the ceiling. Pulse up and down for approximately 1 minute.

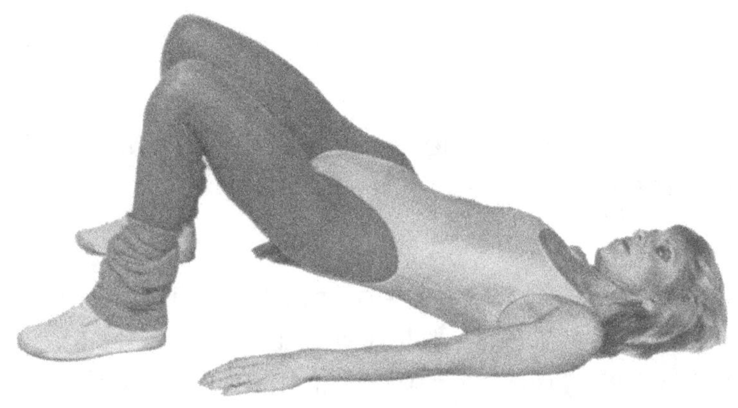

5. BASIC PELVIC TILT (right)—You are in the same position as the BASIC PELVIC TILT, but press upward towards the ceiling with just the right hip. Press off the right heel and squeeze your gluteals as you press upward towards the ceiling. Keep your knees apart. Pull in your abdominals. Pulse upward for approximately 1 minute.

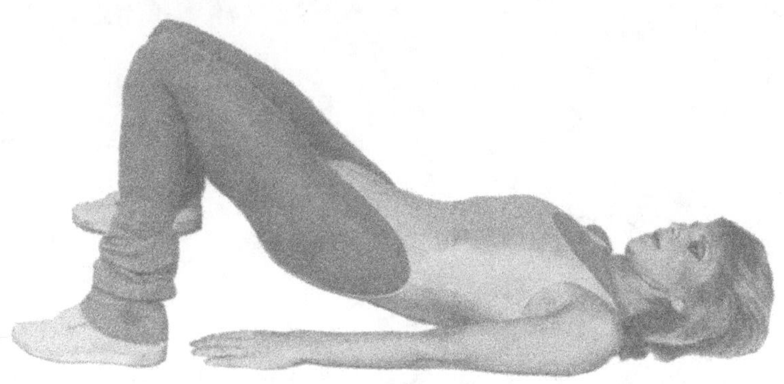

6. BASIC PELVIC TILT (left)—This is the same as #5, but this time press towards the ceiling with your left hip. Press off the left heel. Do this for approximately 1 minute.

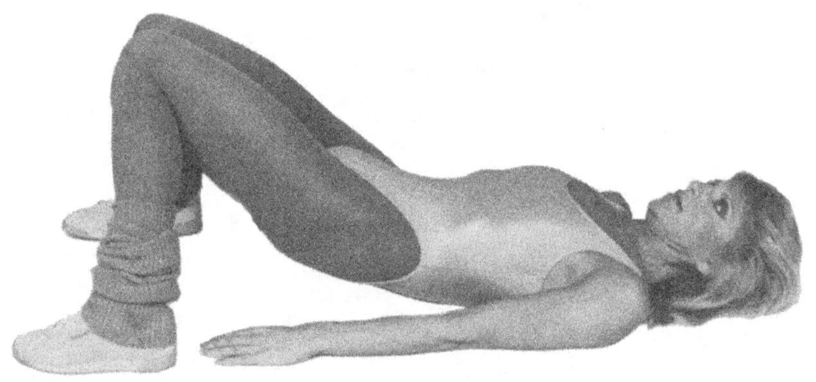

7. STREET DEFENSE—Stay in the same position as the PELVIC TILT, but squeeze your knees together and have your toes turned slightly inward. Do this for approximately 1 minute.

8. OPEN TILT BOOGIE—You are still in the same position as the PELVIC TILT, but turn your toes outward, and have your legs apart. Press up to the right and then to the left. Alternate pulsing right and left for approximately 1 minute.

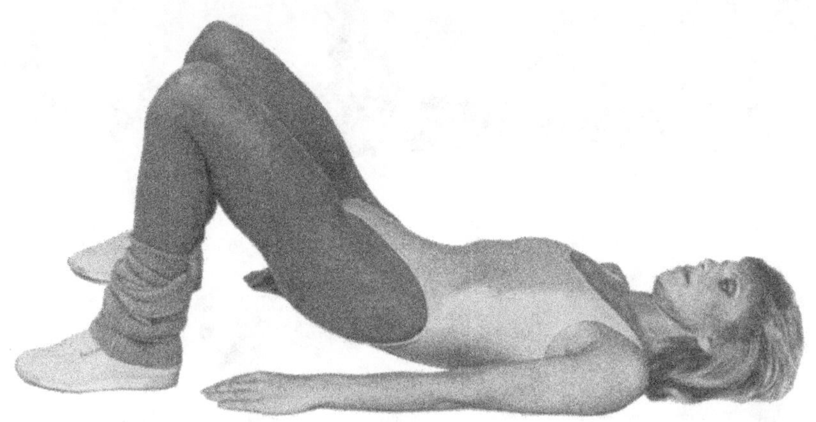

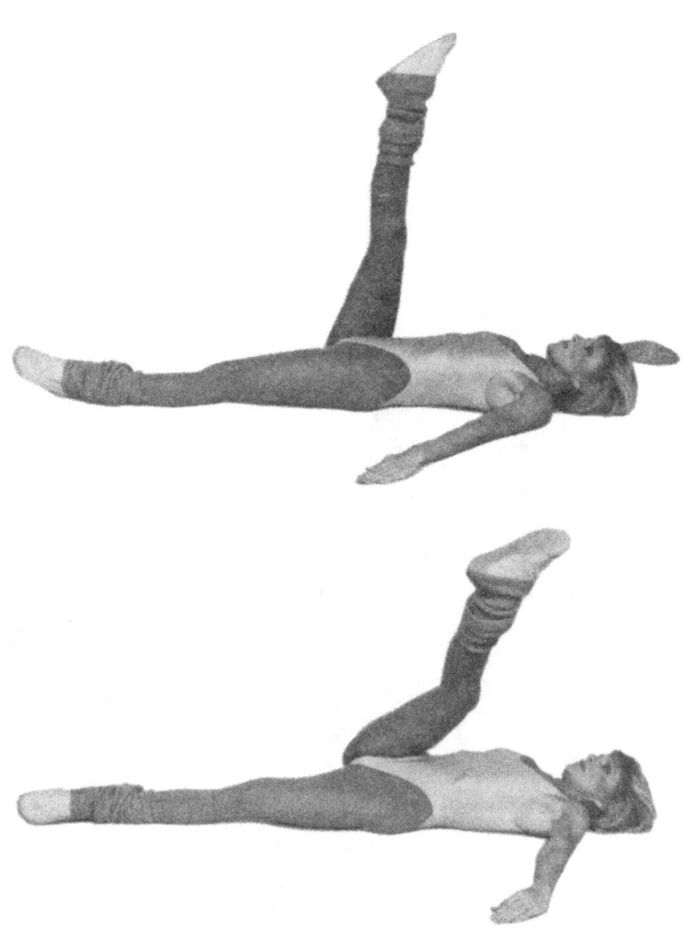

9. UP AND OVER—Lie flat on your back with your arms out at shoulder level. Lift your right leg and cross it over your body aiming towards the left hand. Lead with the heel and try to touch it down. Alternate with the right and left leg. Do this for approximately 1 minute.

10. FANNY FIRMER—Now get onto all fours, and lift your right leg. Bend the right knee and flex the foot towards the ceiling. Press towards the ceiling. Tighten your gluteals, and hold in your abdominal muscles so that there is no strain on your back. Press the foot towards the ceiling for approximately 1 minute.

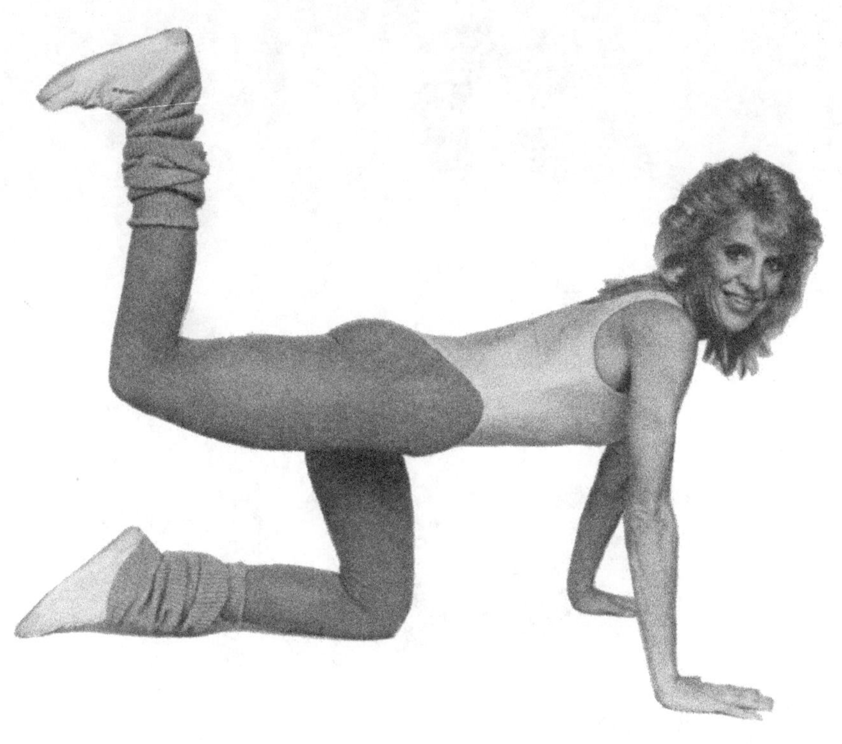

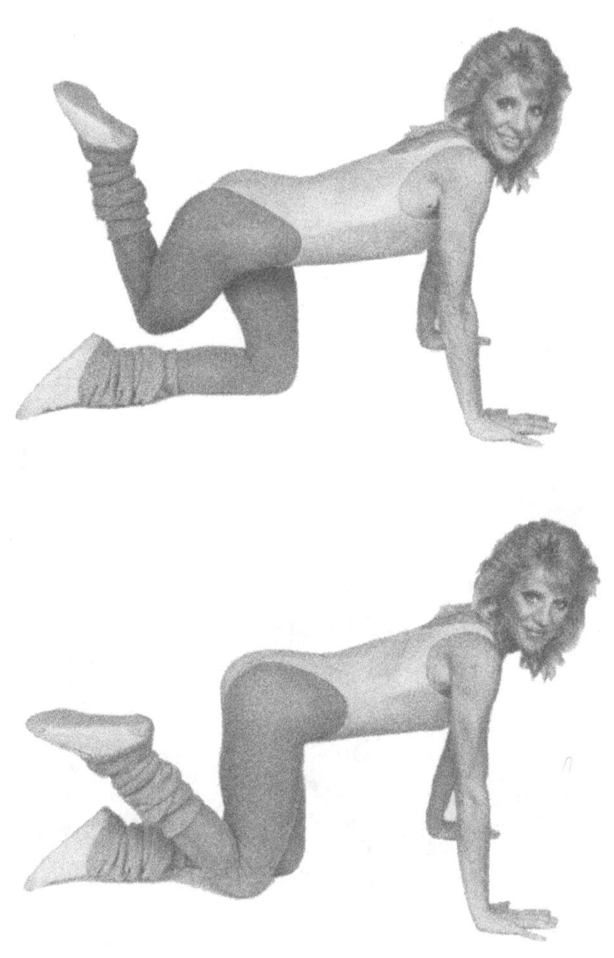

11. FANNY CROSS OVER—Now bring the right knee down to the floor, and bring it up and over the left calf. Lift it up and over for approximately 1 minute.

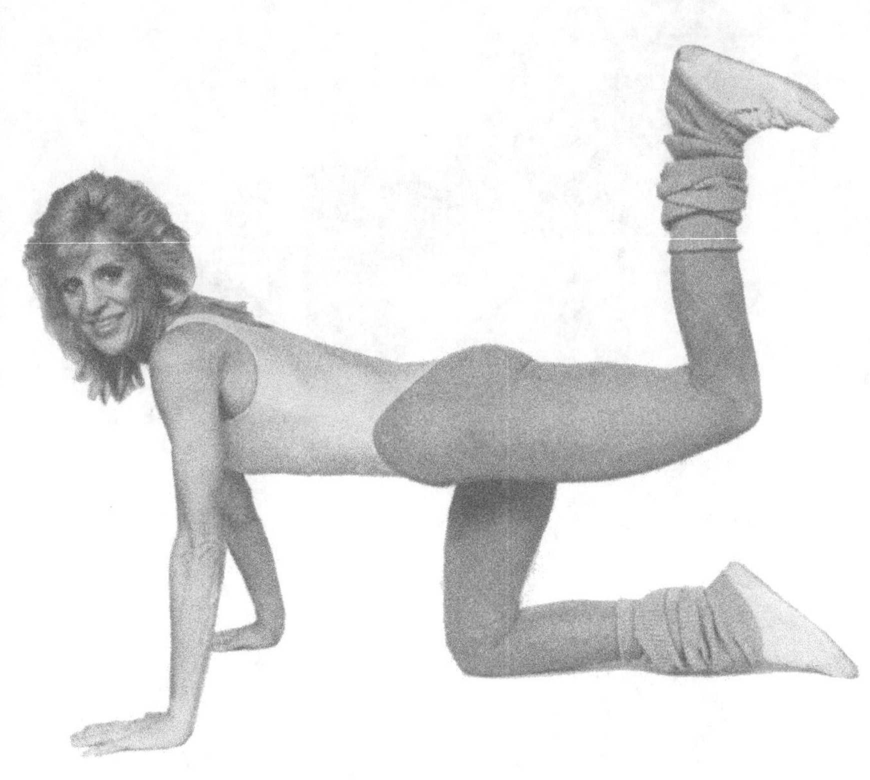

12. FANNY FIRMER—Now get onto all fours, and lift your left leg. Bend the left knee and flex the foot towards the ceiling. Press towards the ceiling. Tighten your gluteals, and hold in your abdominal muscles so that there is no strain on your back. Press the foot towards the ceiling for approximately 1 minute.

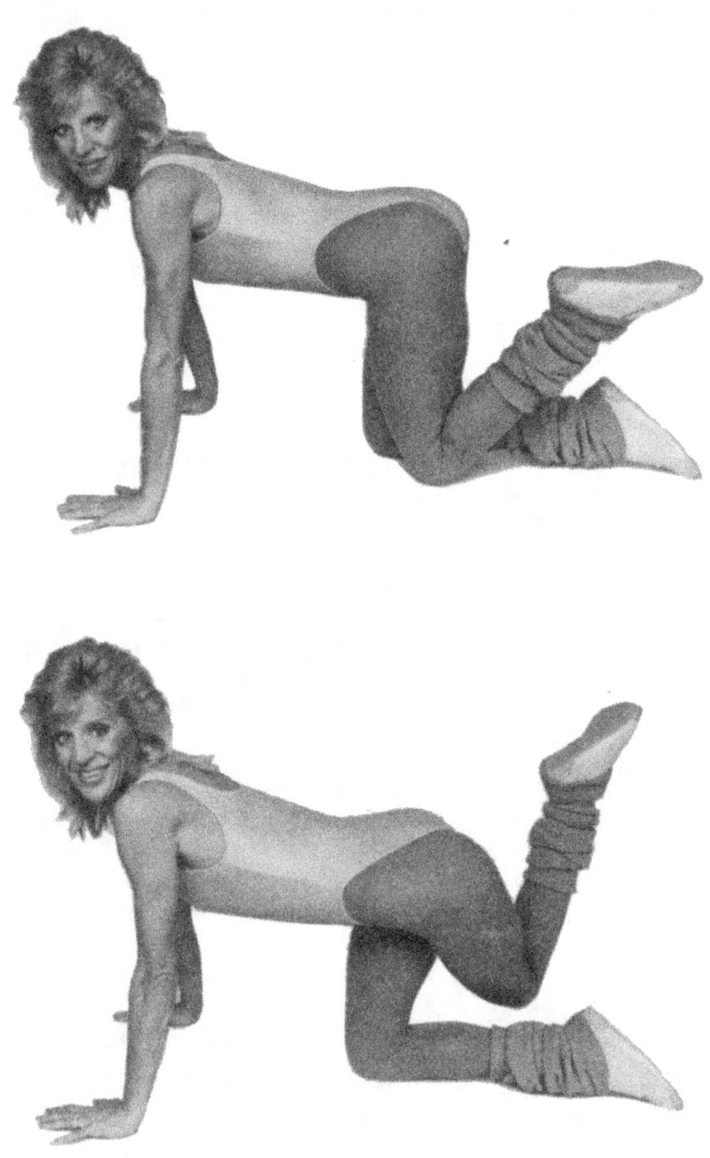

13. FANNY CROSS OVER—Now bring the left knee down to the floor, and bring it up and over the left calf. Lift it up and over for approximately 1 minute.

14. Now roll back, and then roll upward vertebra by vertebra.

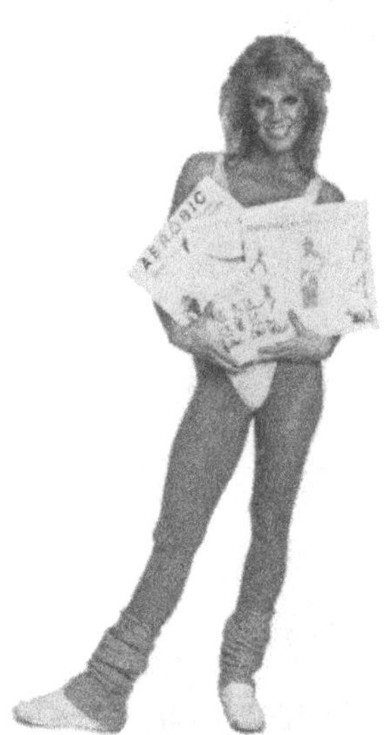

Yeah, you've made it! Feel those FANNY muscles firming. You're going to look great in those new pants. Now, your gluteal muscles might be a bit sore, but that's how you know that your toning, and firming those muscles.

Do this 12 MINUTE WORK OUT at least 3 to 5 times a week, and when you really start getting in shape you might want to repeat the tape two times in a row.

Look for my other 12 MINUTE WORK OUTS to strengthen, tone, and firm other specific body parts.

For a complete work out get my new video tape "Vital, Vigorous and Visual." It's available wherever video tapes are sold. Ask for it by name. Or you may want to consider getting one of my 3 best selling albums. Each one earned a gold record. They are all complete work outs from head to toe. They 're Fantastic! Look and ask for them wherever records or tapes are sold.

Also Available in the The Contoure Fitness Instructional books and recordings/audiobooks series

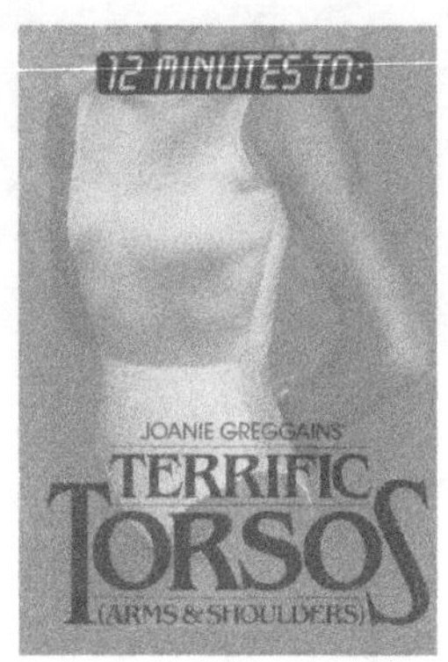

Terrific Torsos

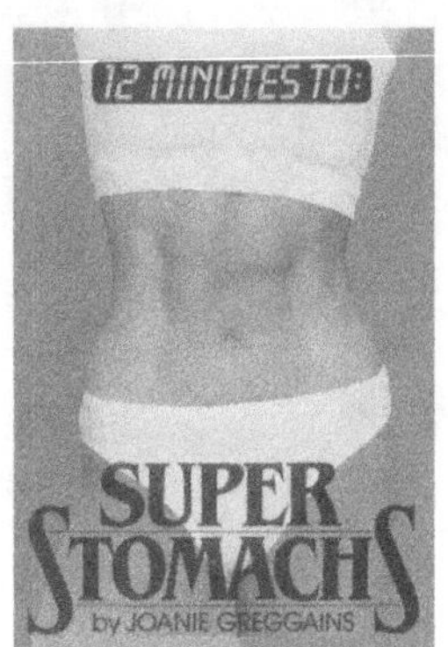

Super Stomachs

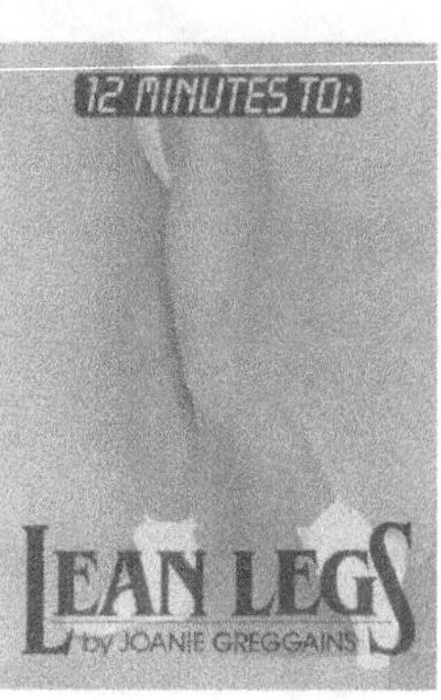

Lean Legs

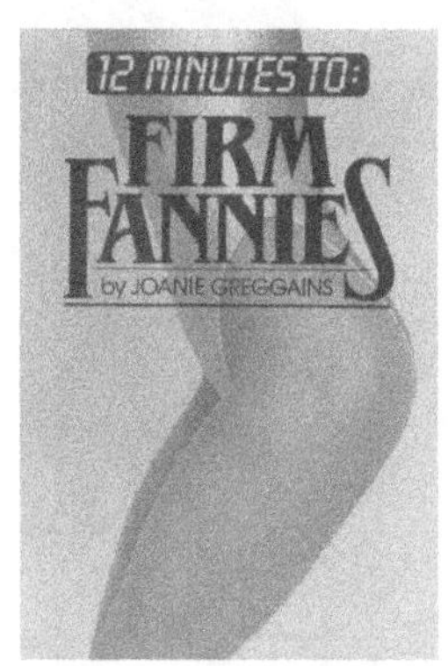

Firm Fannies

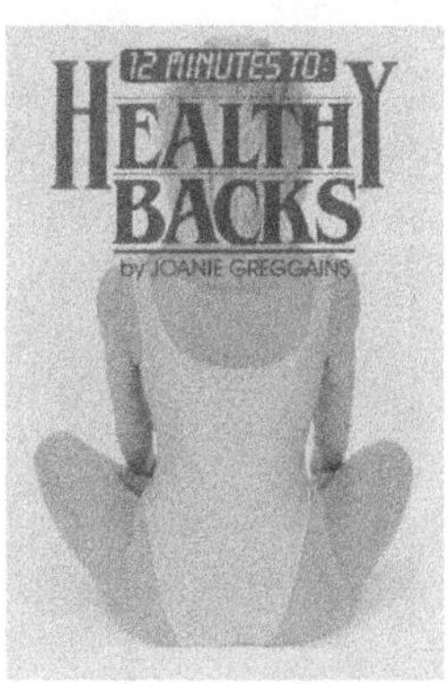

Healthy Backs

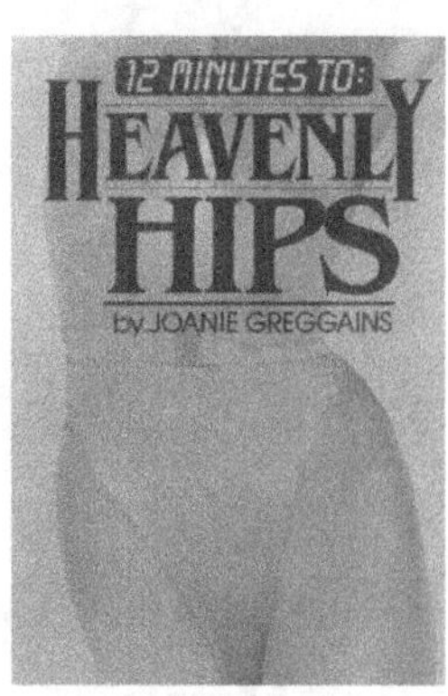

Heavenly Hips

Also Available in the The Contoure Fitness Instructional books and recordings/audiobooks series

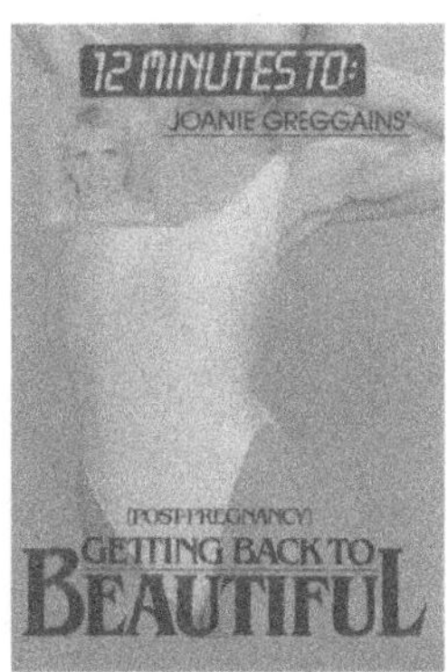

Getting Back To Beautiful

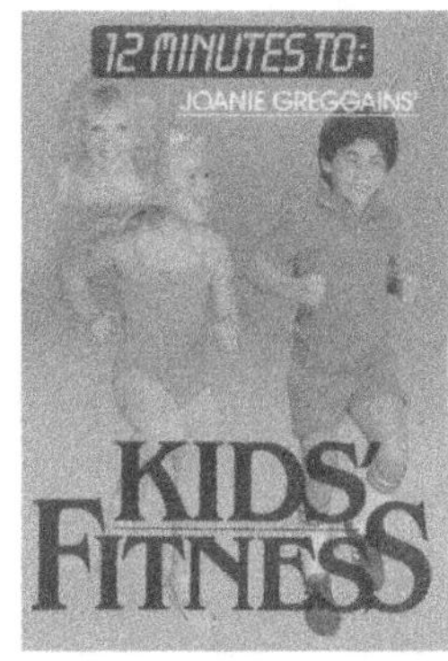

Kids' Fitness

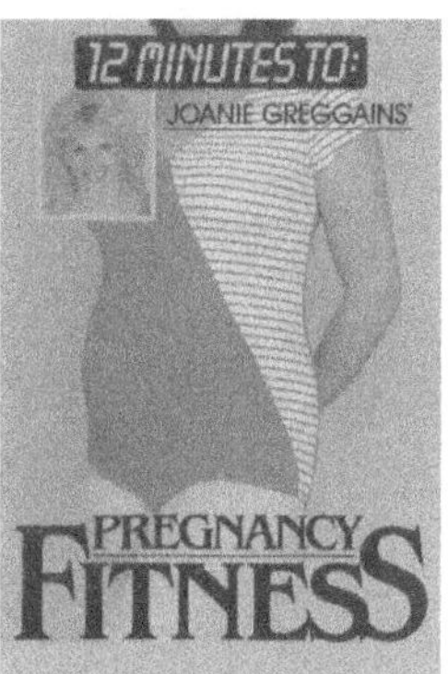

Pregnancy Fitness

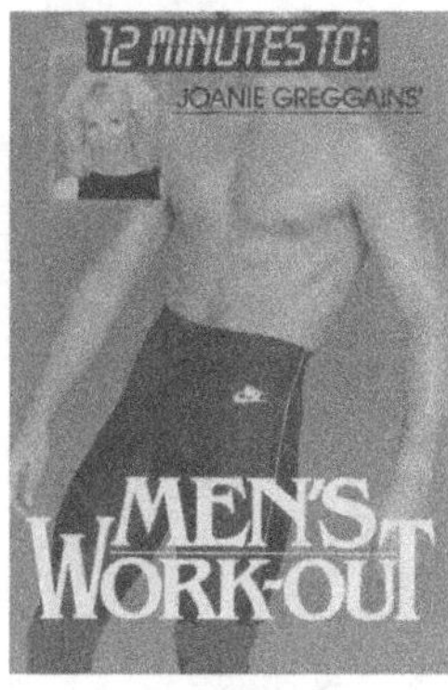

Men's Workout

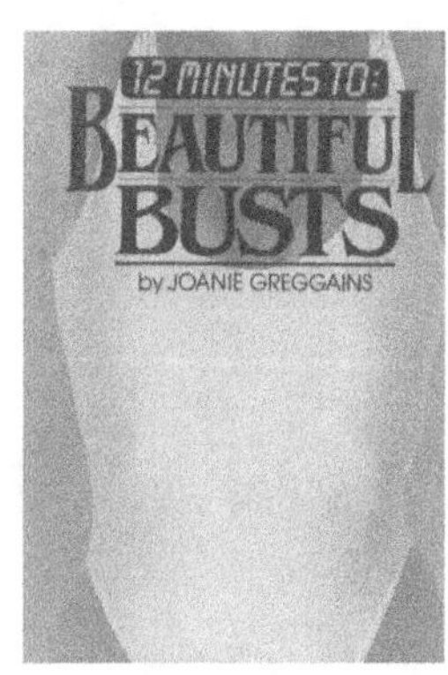

Beautiful Busts

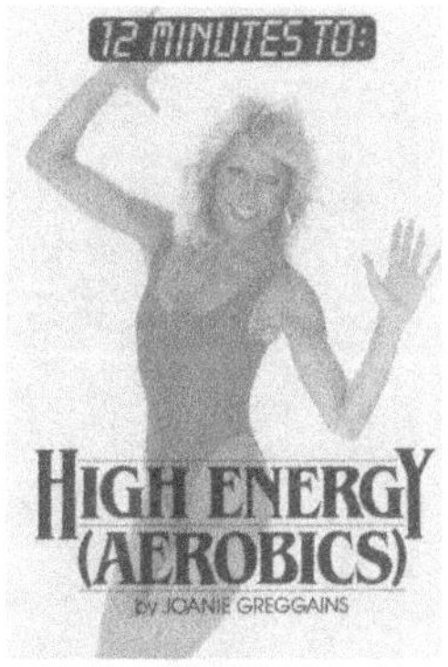

High Energy Aerobics